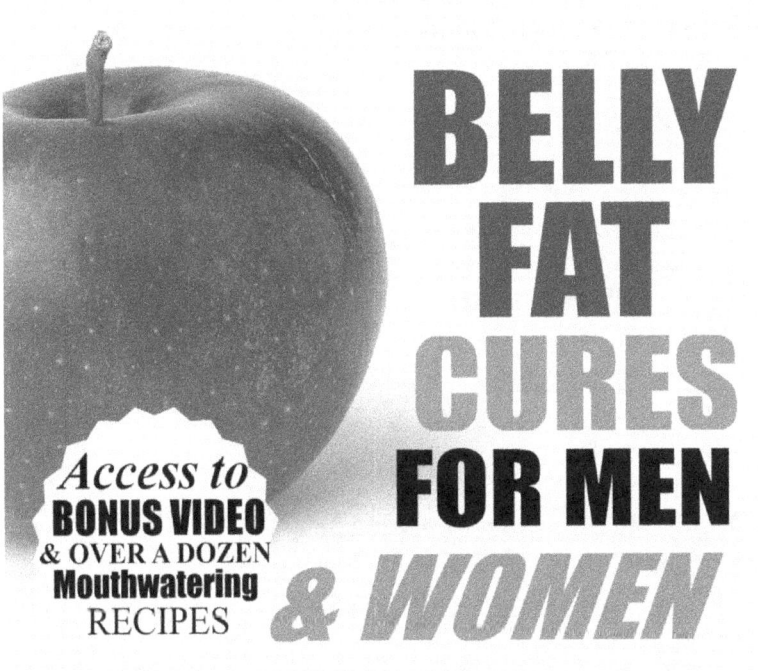

How to Lose Belly Fat Fast and Easy!

BELLY FAT CURES FOR MEN *& WOMEN*

Access to **BONUS VIDEO** **& OVER A DOZEN** **Mouthwatering** RECIPES

Eugene Walker

Powerful Natural Cures And Natural Remedies Revealed

The information contained within **" Belly Fat Cures for Men and Women - How to Lose Belly Fat Fast and Easy"** is based on the author's own experience and research. The sources used for the research are credible and authentic to the best of our knowledge.

In no event shall the author be liable for any direct, indirect, incidental, punitive, or consequential damages of any kind whatsoever with respect to the service or the materials and the products contained within.

Table of Contents

Chapter 1 – Introduction - How to Lose Belly Fat for Men and Women

Belly fat is unsightly and unhealthy, and many men and women throughout the world struggle with losing it. Belly fat is not something that you want to have, but because of lack of exercise, unhealthy eating, or other circumstances – it happens.

Since, as we all know, men and women are totally different beings, the reasons for carrying the belly fat will be different for each gender; and the reasons and means for losing it will be different too.

Therefore, if you want to learn how to lose your belly fat, it is highly suggested that you read the following information specific to your gender. There's a lot to learn, so read on.

Do you want to lose the belly fat that just seems to be glued to your mid-section? Are you unsure of how to go about this? Well, you're not alone. Many people want to know the secret of burning off belly fat and keeping it off forever.

But before you can do this, you have to understand a bit more about what belly fat is. You also need to understand why it is so hard to lose. Only then will you be able to make an intelligent, effective diet and exercise plan that suits your belly fat challenge and lifestyle needs.

So, let's get started on this journey and get you the look that you're after. Once you see the end result – you'll be guaranteed to say it was worth all the hard work and determination.

Chapter 2 - What Exactly Is Belly Fat?

Belly fat is extra weight and fat deposit around the abdomen. This deposit occurs in both men and women. Physicians refer to this as abdominal obesity, as you may not have extra weight anywhere else on your body. Belly fat is not confined to particular people, with particular problems – it can affect anyone.

Belly fat is also something that likely causes certain health conditions and diseases such as diabetes, obesity, and cardiovascular disease. When a person consumes more calories than they are able to use up, extra fat is stored in the body. This fat is carried mostly in the belly area.

The belly area is a central point for a lot of fat to accumulate and settle. This means that certain shirts probably do not look their best on you. It also means that you might look and feel somewhat unhealthy. In fact, you probably are not at your best in any facet if your body fat percentage is much higher than it should be.

Why is it so difficult to lose this weight? Perhaps you're not working hard enough between balancing the right amount and type of exercise with the right diet. For older people, this is even a greater challenge, since they tend to have a harder time losing weight in general. Those that are sick or have limited mobility may not be getting the right help they need to make this work either.

Not get enough sleep for those who are over-stressed can also be a contributing factor. The basic guideline for all situations is to focus on the main foods that shrink belly weight, while also incorporating abdomen specific exercises. By doing this, you are guaranteed to reduce belly fat. Even though sometimes this belly fat may be stubborn, this is really what will work. Do not give up!

The next sections of this article will explain more on healthy body fat percentage rates and how the metabolic rate is an important factor when it comes to burning the fat. So, educate yourself on what can be done to become leaner and healthier!

Chapter 3 - Losing Belly Fat for Men

For men, losing belly fat is easier said than done – just ask the men!

There is good news, however. With the right plan and a little motivation, men really can shed those unwanted belly pounds. Many doctors agree that by making healthier food choices, eating smaller portions, exercising regularly, and getting enough sleep, obesity for men could become a much smaller issue.

But here's a cautionary note: Do not fall for those infomercials that promise a leaner, meaner, muscular body in just a week. These programs are not designed to meet the demands of losing weight and staying healthy. Also, these programs are not designed specifically for men that have extra abdominal weight.

So what is it that you should do?

Set out a diet and exercise plan and stick to it! You will not see results if you're not consistent and keep yourself motivated. By not having the support from those around you and keeping up your own motivation, you're not going to be able to shed the pounds.

You need to feel great about the choices that you've made and move forward. No one else is able to make choices and decisions for you about your own unwanted belly fat. After all is said and done, this is your body, and you need to take care of it.

Chapter 4 - Why Men Have Belly Fat

You often complain about the extra weight you're carrying around. Perhaps you did not have this in your 20's, but now you are reaching 40. You want to look the way you once did, but your life circumstances have changed.

As you get older, you tend to acquire belly fat. This could be for many reasons. Perhaps you have belly fat as a result of entertaining clients at work. You tend to have drinks and dinner with your clients throughout the week. Drinking alcohol and maintaining a poor diet can lead to putting on that extra weight around the mid-section. Then again, maybe you're just sitting at a desk all day long.

If you're not getting enough activity throughout the day, you can easily accumulate that extra weight as well. What if you've had a long day and you just want to sit on the couch when you get home? That's not going to help your mid-section, either.

Maybe you're one of those men who just like to eat – and you enjoy it a lot! In fact, you're ready to enjoy your food all over again, even after you've cleared your plate off the table. Remember how you used to love drinking beer? Well, as you age, that beer sticks to your mid-section. It doesn't process the way it used to when you were younger and only drank socially

So, whether you are out for the night with clients, sitting at your desk while working, or just doing daily stuff, create a viable plan and stick to it. By making your own plan, you're able to personalize every feature. You can design the exercise and meal plan that suits you perfectly.

Even if you're getting older, it doesn't mean that you cannot lose the weight. It just means that you have to work a bit harder to shed the pounds. Do not be one of those men who give up trying. You're really able to lose the belly fat – you just have to get into a new and healthier lifestyle and make it work.

Chapter 5 - Your Metabolic Rate

Your metabolic rate has a lot to do with how much fat you burn. Usually, when you're younger, this rate is much higher than when you're older. That is why a lot of people do not get the belly fat until they have hit a certain age. This age depends on the person. In the case of children, some just have larger body types, poor eating habits, or get minimal exercise throughout the day. This leads to child obesity. Those that were once skinny little children might now be faced with a gut they would rather not have.

This is a combination of diet, exercise, and unbalanced metabolic rate. In order to understand how to reduce the belly fat, you have to understand your metabolic rate. From there, you can move to setting up a healthier diet and incorporating the right exercise into your daily routine.

There is a resting metabolic rate, that refers to your body burning burn fat while sitting, relaxing, and even watching television. Then there is something known as the basal metabolic rate. This is when you check your rate when you have not eaten anything for a day. This measurement tends to be less accurate as compared to the resting metabolic rate – because you do not fast before calculating what it is.

Keep in mind that your resting metabolic rate will slow down as you age. This can be checked to determine what the rate is at any given time. Here are the calculations that are needed to determine your resting metabolic rate:

Your Resting Metabolic Rate = [(6.25 x Weight in Pounds) + (12.7 x Height in Inches) - (6.76 x Age) + 66] x 1.1

The amount that you're left with at the end of this equation is the number of calories that you burn on a regular basis. This includes the food that is currently being digested in your system.

In order to provide yourself with the numbers that you need to lose that belly fat, you have to consume enough calories to cover this. You should not be going over the amount needed since this can cause overeating. That extra food will just sit in your system and become fat – and this fat is what you're trying to lose.

The resting metabolic rate does not account for calories that you burn during physical activity. So, after completing your exercise routine, you may want to have a snack or two just to have those extra calories that you can burn. If you do not have enough calories to burn in your system, you may become tired and have limited energy.

Chapter 6 - Why Is the RMR So Important to Know?

If you're trying to lose your belly fat, it is important to know these figures. They will help you fully plan your diet and exercise plan, since they chart important numbers for you to be able to understand how your body processes food.

The numbers can also help you maintain your current body weight and lifestyle, if you so choose. If you've tried everything but do not seem to be losing weight, then you might be missing something. That something could be your resting metabolic weight number.

Write down your resting metabolic rate and keep it with you. Count your calories if needed. Make sure to stay on track. If you're not hungry, then do not eat extra food. Try finding a hobby that takes up your spare time. It can make a huge difference.

So, how does your RMR come into play regarding your ideal body fat ratio? How can you calculate your body fat ratio and become generally healthier? Read on to find out more.

Chapter 7 - Ideal Body Fat Ratio

Everyone has body fat – but did you know that there is an ideal range for this? Having some body fat is good, but when there is too much, it can be a problem. Find out where you want to be. You can then set a realistic goal to achieve the specified numbers that will give you a healthier weight.

Here are some general guidelines that come along with the ideal body fat ratio.

According to the American Council on Exercise, these are the guidelines for the average male:

- 2-5% for essential fat
- 6-13% for athletic men
- 14-17% for men in shape
- 18-24% for an average weight
- 25+% is considered obese

By finding out what your body fat ratio is, you're able to see where you stand in terms of your overall health. A little fat is good. It can help your essential organs function; it can also heat your body when the temperature is below comfort level. Without the fat, your body will have nothing to burn on a daily basis.

Too much fat, however, can lead to serious health problems, such as diabetes, high cholesterol, and heart problems. With the normal body fat percentage rates, you're way better off than being in an obese state.

So, how do you know what your body fat ratio is? In order to see where you stand according to this chart, you have to know how much fat you have. Keep in mind that height and age also come into play when considering body fat ratios. Adjust the amounts a few percentages higher if you're older or lower if you're younger. Here is a calculation for you to use to find out what your body fat ratio is and where you stand according to the chart.

(1.20 x BMI) + (0.23 x Age) - 16.2 = Body Fat Percentage

Once you figure out your body fat percentage, you can then compare it to the equation above. Are you a little over the normal percentage? A lot over it? If you are, you can improve with good diet and an appropriate workout plan. This plan should help you shed pounds and also turn some of your fat into muscle.

It is important to know your body fat percentage. It is also important to know if you are obese. If you are, it means that you're considered unhealthy. But you can improve your health, improve your weight, and feel and look much better with the right plan.

Chapter 8 - What to Eat

A diet plan should be followed to ensure that you're losing weight and to track the process. However, keep in mind that you have to eat to lose the weight you want. You can't just stop eating, since your body needs calories to burn while working out and doing your daily activity.

If you do not eat, you might shed pounds, but you'll be losing muscle mass at the same time. Not only will eating more healthfully help you lose weight, but it will accustom you to better eating habits.

Stock up your fridge, freezer, and cupboards with healthy, nutritious, wholesome foods. Fruits, veggies and meat should be the essentials. Not only do they provide vitamins and minerals, but they can give essential calories as well. There is a difference between good fat and bad fat, good carbs and bad carbs. You just have to know the differences and know when to say 'no' to certain foods.

Say No to Filler Foods

All fast food is processed food. Think of it as 'filler food.' You're not going to be able to get much value out of the food that your body is not able to use. The food will keep you full, but it will slow you down. Cutting fast food out of your diet is the healthiest thing you can do for yourself.

Soda, beer, and other carbonated drinks are also detrimental, since they contain a lot sugar and fat. Neither this fat nor the sugar is good for your body. By cutting down or eliminating these drinks, you'll be doing your body a great service.

Think Healthy, Be Healthy

It is essential to keep a positive attitude. You need to know that you are what you eat. Those greasy hamburgers are going straight to your gut, and it shows. Now is the time to consider setting boundaries for yourself. If none of your friends are dieting or exercising, well, so what! Go ahead and set an example.

You want to be the one that is out there working towards a goal. If you want to have a slimmer belly, work for it. If you want to be healthier, go for it. It is all about the way you think about challenges and how you're able to take them on.

So, what are some foods that you can eat?

Chapter 9 - Foods That Are Good for Losing Belly Fat

Here is a list of some of the best foods to help curb that belly fat and get you back on track. Remember, stick to the diet plan and make sure to follow your exercise routine to get optimum results. If you get off track, get back on it the next day. Keep trying!

- Milk
- Eggs
- Oatmeal
- Whole grain bread and cereal
- Whole grain pasta
- Berries
- Brown rice

- Nuts
- Hot peppers
- Fruits and vegetables
- Green tea
- Legumes
- Lean chicken, turkey, beef, and fish

Any food that has high fructose corn syrup or other additives is not going to help you. Try obtaining your fruits and veggies from a farmer local to the area. You want delicious, fresh foods to provide the energy you're after.

Not a big vegetable person? No problem!

Try juicing the vegetables. Add in a few fruits for extra flavor. Juicing is a great way to get your required servings of vegetables, while also obtaining the nutrients. You can drink the juice while on the go. Keep in mind, however, that fruits lose a lot of nutritional value when they are juiced, while juiced vegetables are still able to provide their original nutritional value.

Also, many bodybuilders state that by adding a protein powder or other supplement to the juice, you're able to make your own slimming body pre- or post-workout drink.

Here is a list of recommended supplements to increase the nutrients and flavor to an otherwise bland drink that you throw together. Do not forget to grab a juicing book! It has numerous recipes that can give you delicious drinks and take the guessing out of what might taste good when you throw it together.

- 7-Keto to boost your metabolism
- Forskolin to break down fat in the body
- Caraway seeds to beat bloating before it starts
- Relora to reduce stress
- Protein powder for a boost of energy

What about the 'right kinds of food' that you should be eating? Is there a list of foods or a specific food program to follow? Not really, but there are some guidelines and some great belly shrinking foods that you can incorporate into your diet plan. Read on to learn more.

Chapter 10 - Tips for Eating the 'Right' Kinds of Food

Eating food that can help your metabolism is always a winning situation. Carbs are your friends here, so stick with a diet that provides good carbs to burn. You should consider some wholesome meals that are rich in vitamins, nutrients, fiber, and other great extras.

Without these foods, your body is not going to have anything to work with. This is one of the most important steps that you should take. Not only are you making your body healthier, but just by changing your diet, you'll lose those pounds off your waist.

Amount of Food

You might want to stick with the low carb, calculated food diet, but if you're working out, you're going to tire faster. Food is essential for providing your body with something to process and turn into energy. The better the food, the better your energy levels are going to be. Wholesome grains, breads, cereals, fruits, veggies, and lean meat are all critical to your diet. Each has good carbs that your body is able to use.

Eat smaller, more frequent meals. When you eat a large meal, you're not letting your body absorb the nutrients. By eating smaller meals – how about a small bowl of cereal and later on a piece of melon? – you're helping your body slow down, absorb, and then use the nutrients. Bigger is not always better, especially when it comes to eating and trying to burn that belly fat.

So, pace yourself throughout the day. Skip that large dinner or lunch. Opt for smaller portions. Go out to eat less frequently. Make the most out of your meal and enjoy it. You want to make sure that eating is something you like to do, not something you have to do.

Vitamins and Minerals

When choosing foods, choose those that have high vitamin C content. Vitamin C is able to restore and repair the body, and is also responsible for turning fat into muscle. Your fat is not going to be able to go anywhere if your body does not have enough vitamin C. Some of the vitamin C rich foods include kiwi, oranges, kale, and chili peppers.

Do not skimp on your daily protein intake, since the protein provides the building blocks for your physical strength. Your body will need this protein to give you the stamina for your workouts and daily physical activity. Some of the foods that are protein rich include cottage cheese, fish, eggs, meat, whey, and poultry.

Take a probiotic every day. The probiotic is a bacterium that stays in your digestive system, and breaks down and uses the food you eat. Without these bacteria in your body, you're not fully using the food you eat to your advantage. Without enough of the bacteria, you may also get frequent stomachaches. Some foods, such as yogurt, act as a probiotic, or you can find it as a supplement.

Vitamins and minerals are important for weight loss, but also to make you feel better overall. When you eat more healthfully, you're able to get lots more out of life and can become a happier person. Sure, you'll lose those extra pounds, but your body will work better as a whole. Each bodily system will improve over time.

Chapter 11 - What Foods You Should Try to Avoid

There are many things that you should avoid since they may be harmful to your health, but they will also prevent you from losing the mid-section fat. You want to make sure that you go about your weight loss in a healthy manner. Try dropping some of those old habits that you once loved. Don't worry, you will be okay.

Sugar is the enemy when it comes to planning your meal. Don't get caught up in how good it tastes; it is simply bad for you. A lot of processed foods contain loads of sugar. This sugar is actually what is going to build the fat in your body, as it works against you.

So, eliminating the amount of sugar, if not removing it from your diet entirely, can make a significant difference. Alcohol is another item that can contribute to belly fat. Having a drink every now and again can be fine.

Men who drink in excess tend to have large bellies and man boobs. This is not your ideal image, is it! By eliminating alcohol, you're allowing your liver to do the job it is supposed to do, as it cleans out the toxins. Without removing the toxins, your body retains them and turns them to fat. You're also feeling sluggish and sicker.

Tobacco products can make you sick. They can cause you to keep your current weight, or even make you gain weight. Tobacco is known as an appetite suppressant, but it can also depress you, make you eat more, and make it hard for your body to repair itself.

Even if you choose to change your diet and exercise plan, you're still going to have a hard time if you smoke. So, think about kicking this habit to the curb. Speak with local government offices. Many of them have programs for smokers who are looking to quit. Try sugar free gum or busying yourself with a hobby. Quitting might be hard, but it can be done!

Eating out or eating fast food is a bad choice. You need to limit these activities. You can go out once a month, enjoy a healthy menu option, and then go home and resume your plan.

However, if you are eating out very often, or grabbing a lot of fast food on your lunch breaks, this needs to stop. You're not doing your body any favors. It might taste good, but you'll regret eating those foods when you have another look at the belly fat in front.

Now is the time to consider making a new meal plan. Prepare your lunch at home instead of buying it every day. Think healthy with each and every meal that you prepare. By doing this, you're allowing yourself to create better eating habits overall. Skip the Snickers bar and grab a piece of celery instead.

Wondering what a meal plan for a man looks like?

Example Meal Plan for a Day

Breakfast

- Oatmeal with one fruit
- Glass of milk

Snack
- Whole grain peanut butter sandwich
- Handful of berries
- Green tea

Lunch
- Whole grain pasta
- Glass of water
- 3 hardboiled eggs

Snack
- 1 piece of fruit or vegetable

Dinner
- Lean meat of your choice
- Potatoes
- Vegetables
- Glass of water

Snack
- Cup of milk
- Handful of nuts
- Cup of yogurt

You should drink water throughout the day and replace your sugary drinks. This way, you're replenishing your body's water supply. The more water you drink, the better you will feel.

A lot of problems within the body start because a person does not consume enough water throughout the day. You should have at least eight, 8 ounce glasses of water each day. That will make a real difference to how you feel.

Chapter 12 - Exercises to Do

Once you've gotten your meals in order, it is time to address exercising. By integrating exercise with proper meal plans, you're helping your body lose the weight faster. That weight you used to carry will quickly become old news.

Exercise is important. Not just for those that are overweight or have just a little to lose, but for everyone, of any age and from any background. Doing exercise will keep you healthier and more fit. Many men consider bench pressing and lifting weights as their way to exercise.

While this will build stronger muscles, it is not the best for losing fat. So what is good for losing fat? Many men ask this question, but there is no right or wrong answer – everyone is different. However, there are some ways that you can go about losing the mid-section sag and getting tighter abs.

The answer is not crunches. Sure, you're able to do these after you've lost the weight. But doing these before losing the weight, you'll just be tightening the abs – not getting rid of the fat.

Think of the many other ways that this fat can be dropped. There are a lot of other exercises that are actually more enjoyable than the regular crunches that you're trying out.   Check out some of the exercises that are recommended for men wanting to lose their belly weight.

Be Versatile in Your Workouts

If you are strength training, include some cardiovascular exercises like lifting weights and sprinting. Do cardio workouts each day, and strength train every other. Being versatile and committed to weight loss is one of the biggest components of being able to lose belly fat, or any other unwanted pounds.

Here is an ideal, versatile workout session for a middle-aged man:

Visit the gym three times a week. You can increase or decrease this time, depending on your personal schedule and your workout needs. Strength train for two of those three days. Do an hour of strength related exercises such as bench pressing, lifting, pull-ups, push-ups, and lunges.

Once you've done your hour, cool down for a few minutes. Go to the cardio section and run sprints for 20 minutes. On the third day of your exercise regime, do a full hour of cardio. You can follow this up with 20 minutes of strength training. Always make sure to rest and cool down between exercises.

* Less exercise and gym time may be required for those men who are older, unwell, or have disabilities. The important thing is to know your limits and adjust your workout accordingly.

The combination of cardio and strength training, and timing your exercises evenly throughout the week, provides excellent results. Pair this exercise program with your new, healthier eating habits and you'll find that you not only look better, but feel better.

Want some more belly fat burning exercises? Here is a list of the top 10 belly fat burning exercises for men.

1.   Lifting free weights for 40 minutes a day. You can do more or less, alter the weight amount, and then challenge yourself.

2.   Swimming is a great way to burn fat, plus it is fun! Do free swim for an hour and burn hundreds of calories.

3.   High activity sports help burn off a lot of the unwanted weight. You can have fun and be exercising at the same time. There's basketball, tennis, racquetball, and other sports...

4.   Walking provides you with the power to lose that mid-section weight. Remember to swing your arms and keep your muscles tight and tucked throughout the entire exercise. This will help to build your muscles and burn the fat.

5.   Dumbbell side bends are also great to work out the belly area. Grab a dumbbell in each hand and work smoothly from side to side. Move in up and down motions. You should feel your sides burning and working. This is you burning the fat and working the muscles.

6. Do not do crunches. This can lead to a lot of other problems throughout the body, such as neck and shoulder pain, or lower back pain. You're not helping the belly fat problem by doing 200 crunches. You are just adding many other problems to the list.

7. Try an exercise class for strength training and cardio. By combining these two you can have the ideal exercise program while having fun and losing weight.

8. Try doing your exercises in short bursts instead of all in one go. You can then rest your body and keep going. These short bursts help your body lose the weight and gain muscle mass.

9. Planking is a great way to work more than the abs. Hold yourself up in a push-up position with your elbows on the ground. This can strengthen not only the abs (suck them in!) but also your legs and arms.

10. Work more than one muscle group. If you're just focusing on your abs, you're not going to get the best results. By working more than just the abs, you can have a slimmer, more toned appearance overall in a shorter amount of time.

Now that you've read through all the material presented, rest easy. It can be done. Many people before you have lost the extra pounds. The exercise and diet program may seem hard, but if you're really committed and want to lose that extra weight, there is nothing to lose – except that extra belly fat, of course.

Chapter 13 - Ideal Exercises for Men

Here is a list of some of the exercises that are recommended for men. They provide you with a way to work out all of the muscle groups, while still being able to slim the tummy.

This is something that just about anyone is going to love. The exercises are fun to do and you can feel the burn each time you do them. Don't worry – the burn means that the exercises are working.

- A workout known as bicycles can provide you with a way to burn the mid-section fat. This workout requires that you bend over, touch the ground with your hands, and keep your feet moving continuously – much like you're riding a bicycle. This works out the ab section and your arms and legs while incorporating a cardio into the mix.

- Dumbbell roll out is where you slightly arch your back, grab your weights with each hand, roll them in towards you, then back out. Make sure to tuck your belly in throughout the entire workout. You should feel the burn in many different areas. Make sure to use smooth motions. You can stand up on both your legs, or bend one leg and alternate between the two to hold yourself upright.

- Dumbbell front squats provide power in the upper body and around the waist area. Make sure to bend completely. Support the bar using your shoulders and upper body, but maintain your posture and entire self with your core – your abs. Each squat you do also works your butt and your legs.

- Chin-ups are a popular choice for many. They are easy to do since they require little form and are not complicated. All you have to do is grab onto the bar with your knuckles facing outwards. Then use your arm and abs to pull yourself up. Challenge yourself and see how many you're able to do in a few minutes. Make sure to stop and rest between sets.

- Try out a reverse crunch instead of the plain crunches. The reverse crunch provides more power to the core of your abs. You just lay flat on your back with your legs pointing upwards in a 90 degree angle. From there, push yourself up using only your abs.

This will create a burning sensation in the area, and this means the muscles are working. If want a little more of a challenge, lift your legs entirely up. Put them as straight up as they can go. Then put your fingers behind your ears and lift.

So, what are you waiting for? Try some of these exercises today and set up your goals! Be consistent and you'll see results.

Chapter 14 - Tips for a Smaller Belly

There are many tips to remember. Primarily, though, it is key to understand that combining exercise and diet, and working on body fat percentages and metabolic rates, you're able to lose the belly fat effectively and quickly. You will feel and look better almost immediately, and see results once you've gotten into a routine.

Here are some tips:

•   Even while out with the boys, order something healthy off the menu. Do not try to overdo it. You might have one night of fun, but you still want to stay in your routine. This is important for any person to remember. All it takes is one slip to get back to old habits – which is not what we are trying to do.

•   Make sure that you eat your food at least 3 hours before sleeping. You want to give your body enough time to digest, use, and then burn off the food that you ate. When you eat right before bed, you're not burning enough calories to rid your body of what you just ate. This can lead to fat deposits building overnight.

•   Work out together with a partner instead of on your own. This is something that a lot of people might not think about doing. When you work out with someone, you are more motivated to continue the activity. Without a partner, you are likely to quit after twenty minutes. Challenge yourself and have someone with you to keep you going.

•   Eat slower and enjoy your food. When you eat slowly, your body is able to absorb nutrients more efficiently. All too often people are in a hurry when they eat, so the body is not getting all of the nutrients that the food has to give. This can result in many different problems.

•   Stay away from MSG. This is an artificial flavor enhancer that can make you feel full, but only for a limited time. MSG contains no nutritional value. Leave it off your food intake, and go for a fresh fruit or vegetable instead.

•   Limit the amount of electronics that you use on a daily basis. When you're sitting at your computer, watching television, or just playing around on your phone, you're not getting exercise and you're not using your time efficiently. Get out there, make friends, do something! The whole world is in front of you. Grab it and use it to your advantage!

- Fiber is important. It is your friend. Apples, for example, are a good source of fiber and can suppress your appetite longer. After eating an apple, you'll feel full and energized. Foods with fiber all have a lot of nutrients and vitamins. So, whenever possible, eat fiber-rich meals.

By making sure to keep these tips in mind, you set up solid building blocks for your body, your mind, and your life. Use these blocks consistently and keep making progress. Once you've reached your goal, do not stop. You can maintain your new body shape as long as you work hard and stick with the program. It will pay off very quickly and stay that way!

Chapter 15 - Losing Belly Fat – For Women

Women have belly fat problems, too. By addressing the problems, we can understand the difference between how men and women gain and lose weight. Let's take a look at some of the ways women are able to lose their belly fat. You might be surprised at just how similar the methods are to the men's.

Losing belly fat is not something you want to deal with. But if you have it, you're going to want to know how to get rid of it. Maybe you don't feel good about the way you look, or are embarrassed or even depressed because of it. Do not worry, you're not alone. Many women all over the world feel the same way. They feel as if their lives are so busy that they can't worry about the way they look, even if they wanted to.

The good news is that even the smallest change can help you become a better looking, feeling, and healthier you. So, consider the many things that you should and should not eat. We promise you'll still be able to eat some of those things that you love, just in moderation. A small piece of chocolate in the right context is really fine.

Learn more about why you have belly fat and the factors that come into play, and then make the necessary changes.

Chapter 16 - Why You Have Belly Fat

Women tend to get belly fat, really just a small amount around the waist, from eating too much, not exercising, or just from having children. The fat sits under the skin, and it can be unsightly when trying on bathing suits or having to wear a tighter shirt. Also, trying to keep up healthy eating habits while having a baby can be very difficult.

Women put great efforts into how they look and want to lose excess weight as fast as possible. Even if they've had a baby recently, or gained weight for any other reason, they still want to lose the pounds quickly. We all know that losing the weight is important not only to your health, but to how you feel and look.

Belly fat is not a forever thing if you do not want it to be. It's easy to put on, but will take some serious work to get rid of. This does not mean that it is impossible. It just means that you have to pace yourself, take one day at a time, and make sure to set up the best possible regimen to follow.

First consider how much weight you want to lose. Then write that number down – that is your magic number. It should be an amount that allows you to maintain a healthy body weight, as well as a healthy body fat percentage. Stick to a diet and exercise plan that works for you.

Chapter 17 - Your Ideal Metabolic Rate

Understanding the metabolic rate in women is just as important as dieting and exercising. By knowing what you burn on a daily basis – without exercising – you can plan accordingly. Many women do not even consider finding out what they burn each day. But this is a very important factor for weight reduction.

So, what should you know regarding the metabolic rate, and how will it help you succeed in losing belly fat?

Your metabolic rate is a simple calculation that provides you with the number of calories that you burn while your body is in a resting mode.

Your metabolic rate shows how fast your body is able to use the food you eat as energy. This is also something that you should pay attention to while dieting since you do not want to exceed the amount you burn on a daily basis. By making sure to know what your metabolic rate is, you're able to stay under that amount.

So when the time comes to enjoy a meal or a snack, write down how many calories you're eating, then add them up at the end of the day and see just how close you are to your RMR. By adding extra calories during the exercise period, you're also able to increase the amount of fat that is burned off, while also adding energy.

How do you figure out what your RMR is? Here is a quick, easy way to calculate.

Your resting metabolic rate = [(4.35 x Weight in Pounds) + (4.7 x Height in Inches) - 4.68 x age) + 655] x 1.1

This will provide you with an idea of how many calories you burn each day. Keep in mind that these calories are based on how much you burn while sitting or not being active. The amount of calories you burn on a daily basis will increase when your energy level becomes higher. So multiply your RMR by 1.375 for moderate exercise or 1.725 for extremely active exercise. This will give you more of an idea of what to do and how to adjust your eating habits. In all situations, make sure you have all the calories needed to get you through the day.

If you would like to lose the weight around your mid-section, reduce the amount of calories you normally consume on a daily basis. Generally, a 500-calorie decrease is a good start. Being able to maintain your weight is also recommended.

This can be done by watching your ideal caloric intake while resting. Even if you do moderate exercise, keep up with a healthy amount of calories. It is important to understand that calories are necessary for your energy. But if calories are abused, then they also become responsible for the extra weight that you carry around your mid-section.

Also, your husband, boyfriend, brother, trainer, or significant other might have a higher RMR than you. This is normal. Women have a lower RMR, in general, than men. So if your RMR is around 1,600, and you know that a man needs around 2,400, don't panic – these numbers are correct.

Now that you understand a bit more about your metabolic rate, you should feel more confident about designing a diet and exercise plan. You can do it; many people have set this up in the past. Make it work and stick to it.

Chapter 18 - What Your Body Fat Ratio Should Look Like

Body fat ratio is something that a lot of people do not consider. You might know how you look in the mirror, or what the scale says, but do you know how healthy are you? Maybe some of the weight you see displayed on the scale is muscle, and that's okay. But you need to find out more about where your body fat ratio should be and how you can maintain those healthy numbers.

There is a way to calculate your body fat percentage. There is also an ideal body fat percentage especially for you. Depending on your age, height, and some other factors, you might find that you need to reduce the percentage to reach the goal you want.

The American Council on Exercise recommends these guidelines for body fat percentages for women –

- 10-13% of essential fat
- 14-20% for athletes
- 21-24% for fitness levels
- 25-31% for an average built woman
- 32+% is considered obese

While these are good guidelines to go by, age seems not to be considered here. Yet age is something that can make a difference – and the same is true for a person's height. With so many factors that come into play, consider only your own unique situation.

The general rule for women is the younger you are, the less your body fat percentage should be. The amounts range from 18% to 27% for average built women. Of course, with exceptions, there are lean women, above average women, and those who are considered overweight or obese.

To find out what your body fat percentage is, check out this calculation:

(1.20 x BMI) + (0.23 x Age) - 5.4 = your body fat percentage

This is a calculation that can provide a general idea of where you stand. By understanding the importance of this percentage, you're able to get the most from your workout and diet plan. This plan is something that can help you lose some of your body fat percentage, build muscle, and cut down on the belly fat.

What should your diet and exercise plan look like? Many women will diet and exercise, but not actually have any specific goals in mind.

Here is a general idea of what you should and should not be doing for diet and exercise.

Chapter 19 - What to Eat

Even though you love dipping into your chocolate stash, you have to consider some better ways you could be eating. There are many essential vitamins, minerals and other foods you should be eating – those that can provide you with the building blocks needed to burn fat and build lean, mean muscle.

One thing to keep in mind before you start is to keep your caloric intake around the metabolic rate that you have. If you do this, you'll able to shed some pounds really quickly. So calculate where you stand, then choose foods throughout the day that give you these calories, and not too many more.

Eat Smart

Throw out the junk food and think healthy. The better you eat, the faster you're going to lose weight and burn calories. Keep in mind that you have to eat. You have to put wholesome food into your body to ensure that you have something to burn.

Without essential nutrients, you will find yourself losing weight, but still have the extra around your mid-section. Food that is saturated in fat can cause you to gain excess weight. Food that does not provide minerals, vitamins, or other building blocks, cannot be used by the body. By giving yourself food that you can use, you're helping yourself burn the fat.

Eat more food but fewer carbs. Eating bad carbs will actually prevent you from losing weight. These bad carbs are found in the processed and fast food that you eat. Fuel your body with good food, not bad food, without eating a large meal of junk.

Here's an important principle: If you're full – stop eating. You probably already know this, but keep it in mind as a general rule. Many people continue eating even after they are full. This can lead to obesity and certainly is one of the causes of those unwanted bellies. If you listen to your body, actually listen while eating, you're able to cut down on the amount of food that you eat on a regular basis.

The Essentials of Eating for the Nutrients

Protein is one of those essentials when it comes to choosing your food. The more protein, the better. You need to have protein in order to build muscle, while removing fat. Many people don't get enough protein in their daily diet. However, with careful planning, you're able to get it in yours.

Tuna, eggs, milk, whey, chicken breast, and cottage cheese all contain protein. There are also protein supplements available that can provide you with the essential proteins needed for the day. So, make a shake or take it in pill form.

Drinking green tea is something that cannot be stressed enough. Green tea provides you with nutrients and also boosts your metabolism. You can drink it hot or cold. As a bonus, it also tastes great. So why not add this to your diet plan?

When considering dairy products, always choose low fat options. These options allow you to get the nutrients from the milk without all of the added fat. Whole milk, however, may be good for some.

For infants, or those who are underweight, whole milk instead of the thinner varieties is a better option. For adults, choosing low fat milk is always a good idea.

Fruits, vegetables, and meat all provide the building blocks needed to be healthy, feel great, and slim down that waist line. Stop the comfort eating that you do throughout the night.

If you're feeling down, or are just bored, try doing something other than eating to comfort yourself. Read a book, take a walk, or do other activities. Always consider small, healthy snacks if you must, but look for something else to do besides snack if you just need to pass the time.

Chapter 20 - Foods that Help Burn Belly Fat

These foods are able to help you break down that stubborn belly fat. Incorporate them into your meals, or make meals from them to provide you with the essential nutrients.

- Fish
- Cottage Cheese
- Oats
- Grapefruit
- Vegan Soups
- Bananas
- Lentils and Beans
- Lean Meat
- Whey Protein Powder
- Eggs
- Olive Oil – Skip the vegetable oils, since they are full of bad fats that can cause your body to bloat and build unnecessary fat in places that you don't want it.

Bread is something that you can give up. When you do that, you'll notice a huge difference in the way you feel. A sandwich will fill you up, but you're not actually benefiting from it.

Even if you do not give up bread entirely, eating it only once or twice a week can make a difference. Try whole wheat versions instead of white or Italian bread. That too will make a significant difference.

Chapter 21 - What Your Meal Plan Should Look Like

Wondering how your meal plan should look each day? Here are some simple guidelines that you're able to follow. Get an idea of what you can throw together easily. Keep in mind that eating smaller, more frequent meals throughout the day is better than eating larger, less frequent meals.

Snacking two to three times a day in between meals is good to do as well. If you eat a smaller meal for breakfast, lunch, and dinner, you'll have room for a few healthy, small snacks in between meals.

Snack Ideas

- Handful of nuts or berries
- One piece of fruit such as a banana or apple
- Cup of yogurt
- Whole wheat crackers
- Cup of cottage cheese
- Hot peppers

Breakfast Ideas

* Eating protein at breakfast time will give you a boost for the day. Give yourself that little extra boost of energy to make it until your morning snack.

- Cup of hot oatmeal
- Cup of fruit
- Piece of whole wheat toast
- Milk
- Whey shakes

Lunch Ideas

* Eat a light lunch. This can help you go through the day without that tired feeling. It can also lighten you and make you feel better until you get to dinner.

- Peanut butter sandwich on whole wheat bread
- Whole grain pasta
- Vegetable juice
- Green tea

Dinner Ideas

* Dinner doesn't have to be boring. You can spice things up. Try to reduce salt as much as possible, using it only in moderation.

- Lean meat of your choice
- Potatoes
- Vegetables
- Whole grain pasta
- Milk

Drink water throughout the day so you do not become dehydrated. This can become a serious issue when it comes to losing weight. Many people think that drinking water can cause weight gain.

However, without enough water in your system, you won't feel as fresh. The more water you drink, the easier it will be to lose that belly fat. The recommended amount is eight, 8 ounce glasses per day.

You'll be able to achieve more if you plan ahead and make sure to know what you're going to eat throughout the week. Statistics have shown that those who are dieting but do not plan, fail.

Those who have a set plan succeed and also have a healthier lifestyle. You're able to increase your energy, reduce the risk of disease, while also lose that stubborn belly fat. Plan ahead and follow the road to the new you.

Chapter 22 - How Can You Plan Healthy Meals with Kids?

Many women have that middle section of weight as a result of their body's child bearing. First, they carried their babies for nine months, which definitely affected their stomach area. Now, with the children taking up so much of life, there is hardly time for any exercise.

And who wants to prepare an entire meal for just yourself? It's just more work. At the end of the day, you just want to get the chores done quickly, and then get some rest. So, you'll end up eating what the kids eat. It's just so much easier.

Another dilemma for many women is how can they teach their kids to make healthy food choices?

This is a good question. Not only is it beneficial to eat right, but it is important for the kids to eat right too. Healthy habits should be instilled early in life, which means – the sooner, the better. By talking to your kids about these healthy choices, you're setting them up for good eating habits down the road.

Many people are already eating healthfully. They are aware of detrimental chemicals used in food. No one wants to eat fillers and artificial additives. People want wholesome, pure ingredients and want to feed their kids the same. You might already be providing your kids with a well-balanced, wholesome diet, and that's great!

Here are some tips for those of you who have picky eaters at home:

•   Try to make eating healthy fun. Try out different designs, looks, tastes, textures, and other things that make kids interested. The more interested they are in what they eat, the more likely they are to want to eat it.

•   Let them help prepare the food. This gives them a job, keeps them busy, and gets them excited about the food. They will be more motivated to try out the food if they helped prepare it.

•   Try not to give them too much information about what they are going to be eating. They may not want to eat something if someone else says it's 'yucky.'

- If they will not eat vegetables, try some healthy dips. These can be more fun while also give the veggies a different taste. You, however, shouldn't dip. Try to set a good example by eating your veggies plain.

- Introduce new foods gradually. A bite here, a bite there. Maybe a new food with dinner every now and again. They will begin to ask for the ones they like the most.

- Do not restrict food, use it against the kids, or reward them with it. This can lead to eating disorders later on.

- Praise them for eating their food, for making healthy choices, and so on. The kids will appreciate this and be able to focus on what they should and should not eat. Also, do not nag or punish them for not eating what they chose to put on their plate.

- Sit down as a family every night to eat dinner. This is a good rule to live by. Not only can it bring everyone closer, but it can make this a favorite time of day. When everyone is eating the same thing, at the same time – kids are more likely to eat better.

- Keep junk food out of the home. Whatever is accessible gets eaten. When you choose to put healthy snacks in the home, kids are more likely to eat those rather than other substitutes. Plus, if it's not in the home, you'll to stay on track, as well.

Keeping up with good eating habits is good for the whole family. That includes even your husband, boyfriend, or significant other. Making sure that you're a smart leader in nutrition can set healthier ground rules for everyone else involved.

Chapter 23 - Exercises to Do

What about exercising? What should you do when you want to feel great and be as active as possible?

Around 50 percent of your body fat is located right under the skin. This means that it is also on top of the muscles. The average woman is able to do crunches all day long, but not see any results. You're not moving the fat; you're toning your abs underneath it.

You want to provide yourself with an easy-to-follow plan. This plan should be followed throughout the week in intervals. Do not overdo your workout, because what you are doing is actually causing the fat to move in. You're also putting a lot of strain on your body, which is not good, and which can lead to problems later on.

Do not put all of your trust into supplements and promises that you will lose the weight within days or weeks. This is hype and is something that many people really believe. Do not be one of those people. You can create your own plan, be your own person, and find a specific plan and schedule that works best for you.

Have a Good Mindset

When you put yourself in the right mindset, you're able to accomplish a lot more. When you say to yourself that you can do this and see results, you'll move forward and get those results. Without actually being able to feel good about what you're doing, you're not going to feel motivated to actually do what needs to be done.

If you gain a few pounds one week, work extra hard the next week to remove them. It is all about being positive. Be able to sit up tall, increase your posture, stretch often, and feel good about the way you look and who you are. If you do not like your belly fat, the answer is simple – fix it! It all starts with you. You're the one that has to have the motivation to get the look you want.

Feel good about the changes that you're going to be making. It will be worth it in the end when you see the results. Just take it one day at a time.

Chapter 24 - What Your Exercise Plan Should Look Like

When it comes to designing a personal exercise plan, mix things up a bit. You want to ensure that you're working all of your muscle groups and not just your belly area. You're able to lose even more weight when you work all the muscles together. Here is what your workout schedule should look like. Feel free to modify as needed for your own situation and body type.

This is for a middle-aged woman looking to lose extra belly fat.

• One hour of strength training followed by 20 to 30 minutes of cardio. The cardio can also be done before the strength training exercises. You can choose running, walking, swimming, or anything that gets your heart rate up. Do this for three out of seven days a week.

• Devote one day to yoga or other stretching exercises. These can help strengthen your inner core while also relaxing the muscles. It's also good for your overall relaxation.

• One hour of cardio followed by 20 to 30 minutes of strength training. This should be done once to twice a week. Make sure it is on different days than the yoga and not at the hour of strength training.

• One day of rest. Give your body time to heal and rejuvenate after a long week of working out. This is essential for losing the belly fat.

• Make sure that while weight training, you're doing short, intense periods of workout, and then resting. You want to ensure that you get pumped for those minutes that you're lifting. This can help strengthen muscles and decrease weight while burning off the fat.

Chapter 25 - Ideal Exercises to Burn Belly Fat – For Women

There are very many types of exercises out there. Which ones actually work for you? You do not want to spend countless hours doing something that is not going to show results. You also do not want to spend your time doing something you're not going to enjoy.

The workouts you do should provide results, since results are the ultimate goal. And burning that extra belly fat is the goal. Remember that you have control over what to do, what not to do, and how much to do.

Here are some excellent belly fat exercises for women. They are able to help you shed those extra pounds and feel good about yourself. Take a minute and find out which ones you like. Mix them up a bit each week and have fun.

Weight training is a great way to go about toning muscle and losing weight. It is not something that is just for men, either. However, to do lifting, you need proper form to make sure that you're doing the lifting right.

Working with someone who knows about proper lifting, or hiring a personal trainer, will definitely help, and you'll learn something new in the process. Weight training should be paired with cardio. Do not leave it up to the weights alone.

Yoga is an excellent way to feel good inside and out. It can stretch your muscles, tighten and tone your core, and produce all around great results. Yoga classes will teach you the basic moves. You can also rent a DVD or search the Internet to learn how to do yoga at home. Yoga is a wonderful pastime and gives you much more than an exercise.

Walking is underrated. Many people think there is little benefit to walking because it is not high intensity. It doesn't have to be, though. By taking the time to walk during the day, you're able to burn calories and burn them fast.

Imagine, you can get fresh air at the same time! People do not get enough of this. By adding walking to your routine, you're also allowing yourself some cardio that is not too intense.

Want a little bounce in your life? Try an exercise ball. Not only are you working your body and getting cardio – but it is fun! If you do not have an exercise ball at home, you'll find one in the gym.

You can also purchase one inexpensively in different stores. You can actually get a lot out of the exercise ball that can help you burn unwanted belly fat.

Additionally, you can try Tae Bo or other martial arts. These help you strengthen abdominal muscles, while working on other areas. You're also able to learn some pretty cool moves and have a good time.

These workouts are specifically designed for MMA fighters, and women who want to protect themselves and build lean, mean muscle while burning excess weight.

Get some friends or your family members involved. When you work out with someone else, you're more likely to be consistent. When you have your children workout with you, you set a good example for them.

Plus, it takes a lot of the boredom out of working out alone. Many people drop out of their routine because they do not feel like it is worth it or because they just get bored with the whole thing. Don't become one of these. Make it work and make it count.

What about those oblique's? You don't want to worry about losing the tummy weight then discover that your oblique's are still holding on to that extra weight. You want to make sure while weight training that all this works smoothly together.

Make sure to work out all the muscles in your back and waist. This should go along with working out all the other muscles in the body. The obliques are no exception! This is also an area that can look great when you're in a bikini!

Chapter 26 - Women and Water Weight

Women are plagued by many different things during the course of a month – water weight, or bloating, is one of these. Women do not particularly like this extra weight nor the feeling of zipping up jeans in the morning and feeling them tighter than yesterday.

There are things you can do to reduce the amount of water weight that you experience each month. Try some of these helpful tips and see how much your belly fat is able to shrink down.

• Drink more water! It seems contrary to what makes sense, but it really does work. When you drink more water, your body will naturally soak it up. With the body's water content at about 50-75%, you need to replenish it as much as possible. Drink more, not less water, and feel the bloat subside.

• Reduce the amount of salt you consume. Salt tends to add to water weight. If you eat a lot of salty foods, the extra belly fat can increase. Enjoy your food without the extra salt. It's better for you, and you'll get accustomed to different flavors.

• Eat a lot of fiber. This can make bowel movements more regular. It can also ensure that the water weight and belly fat is reduced. By making sure you're regular on a daily basis, you're allowing yourself to become healthier, while also becoming slimmer.

• Eat yogurt. It contains healthy bacteria (a natural probiotic) that can help reduce the water weight. During the time that you're feeling bloated, eat yogurt more frequently. In fact, eating yogurt regularly is a good idea too as it helps break down enzymes, improving digestion overall.

• If you want to use over the counter water pills, remember to speak to your doctor first. You also want to make sure you follow the instructions given on the pack.

Once you have gone through the list of ways to reduce the water weight, try them out carefully. They might help you feel better and even figure out what to do about the belly fat. At the same time, of course, maintain a healthy eating and exercise plan. All this can help you lose pounds, and keep them off.

Chapter 27 - How Your Hormones Play a Part in Weight Gain

Too much estrogen can cause the body to produce unnecessary fat. This is why when women go on birth control; the extra estrogen can make them gain weight. There are choices for birth control that do not contain estrogen, but they are not as readily available.

If you're gaining weight, but haven't changed anything in your daily life, it might be due to your new birth control method. This is something you should speak to your doctor about.

They can prescribe a different birth control method, and can also help you get onto a plan for reducing the estrogen levels in your body. By reducing these levels, to normal levels, you'll be able to lose that extra weight. Consider this when going on birth control.

It might be a good idea to try different birth control methods until you find one that doesn't make you gain weight. There are many options to choose from. You just have to find the one that works best for you.

Speak to your doctor to learn more about the many different birth control options that are available. Make sure to let your doctor know that you're trying to lose excess weight and to lead a healthier lifestyle. The doctor will be able to personalize a birth control method that is right for you.

Chapter 28 - Tips for a Leaner, Healthier You

There are many tips that women can follow to become leaner and healthier. It can take some time to achieve your goal, but it can be done. In addition to eating better, exercising more, and knowing your metabolic rate and body fat percentage, there are some additional things to keep in mind.

• Choose foods that have a low glycemic index. Food is rated on a scale between 0 to 100 for glucose, with 0 being the best and lowest, 100 being the worst and highest. Look for foods that have a rating of 55 or less. That's what you should be eating. These foods include beans and lentils, whole grains, and most vegetables.

• Always make sure that you're on top of your vitamin intake. If you're not getting enough vitamins through the foods you eat, consider taking supplements. This is an important consideration since vitamins are needed to help the body absorb the nutrients... and they are good to boost your energy levels.

• Cut back on the unnecessary things you do or eat. This might sound a bit weird. However, when you're watching television a lot, you're not active. If you're eating junk or fast food all the time, you'll fill up, but not healthfully. Vitamins and nutrients are not naturally part of these foods as they are part of natural foods such as fresh fruits, veggies, and meat.

- Be persistent and stay motivated. You need to believe in yourself and make sure you can do it. If you do not have the drive, you're not going to be able to succeed. Believe in yourself and you will be able to lose the weight easily.

- Manage your stress. The more you become stressed, the more likely you are to eat and the more you'll sit around. You need to feel good each day. The only way to do this is by reducing the amount of stress you have in your daily life. This is much easier said than done, as we all know, but your efforts will pay off.

- Eat dark chocolate. This is a good thing for any woman (or man!). You're able to get much more out of that dark chocolate that you snack on than a bar of milk chocolate. The dark chocolate contains natural fat burners, not to mention less artificial sugar that can be harmful to your health.

- Set an example. Make sure to be a leader, not a follower when it comes to losing weight. That belly fat is able to shrink down, and your friends and family will surely notice the change. You're able to set a strong example for many other people out there that want to do the same. It might also make you feel good to know you've done it on your own.

- Detox your body. It's a great way to cleanse, and can feel really nice. If you're able to visit a sauna, then do so and let the toxins go. You'll feel much more refreshed and have a rejuvenated mind as well. When you cleanse your body, you're able to let go of the oils and other bad elements that have become trapped.

With these tips, you're well on your way to achieving success. Stick to your beginning goals. Keep all this information in mind as you reach for that double cheeseburger. Many women have gone through the journey that was able to change their life. You can become one of those women that changed her life for the better.

Learn about some myths regarding losing belly fat for both men and women. You might be surprised. Are you doing something wrong? Why isn't it working out? Find the answers here and make sure you're not making any of the common mistakes mentioned on the list. You might be working against yourself, if so!

Chapter 29 - Myths about Losing Belly Fat

There are so many things that you should be doing to help you lose the belly fat. But do you know that there are things you shouldn't do, as well? Some things were mentioned earlier, so they may be repeats.

Some of these are new. Keep this page open and remind yourself not to do these things when you would like to shed those unwanted belly pounds.

- You cannot just diet or just exercise. You need to do these together if you want to lose weight. If you eat junk food and then go exercise, you'll defeat the entire purpose. If you eat healthfully but do not exercise then you're not burning any of the unused nutrients.

- You're working out the wrong way. This could be because you have bad form and are just working your abs. Whatever the reason, you need to make sure to find out how to do exercise and make sure you're doing the right ones. Perhaps the workout you're doing is not challenging enough to your body. Remember, you have to push the limits.

- You're not getting enough sleep. This seems like it has nothing to do with losing weight, but it does. If you're not rested enough, you're not going to be able to lose the extra weight that you have. A full 8 hours a night is essential to weight loss.

- If you're overly stressed, you're not going to be losing weight. Pace yourself in everything you do, and take life day by day.

- Not having enough motivation to get through it. This is something that causes a lot of people to quit. Even if you have no one at your side, being able to stay on top the issue is essential. Believe in yourself and what you're able to do.

- No pain, no gain. Even though this is an old, respected adage, it is not necessarily true. You can do workouts without being in pain. You can feel the burn, but if you're in pain – you might want to rethink the way you're doing the exercise.

- Do not go on a fad diet. These tend not to work out for a lot of people. You might not be getting the nutrients you actually need, either. Find your own comfort level with both your diet and exercise by coming up with your own, customized plan.

Chapter 30 - Do Genes Play a Role?

What about those genes? Do you think that they play a role in your body figure? Perhaps the women on your mom's side have a little more to love. Whatever the reason is, learn more about genetics and how they play a large part in the body type you have.

Genes definitely play a significant role in your body type. However, the body is an amazing thing that can be changed. You probably know someone with good genes. They are able to keep their slim figure even after eating 10 Big Macs and 8 large fries.

They might not be the healthiest person you know, but they still are not gaining weight the way you are. That's because your genes are not the same as theirs. You have to ignore your genes and actually work to get the body that you want.

Don't feel helpless. That stuff around your middle can be removed, but it is going to take some time. Work hard, know your goals, and stick to your plan. Not everyone is blessed with the skinny gene, but you can work with what you've got, too.

Chapter 31 - Set Your Own Goals and Plans

Set your own goals for exercise and a diet plan. You can use the examples mentioned here to provide yourself with a general strategy. Just fill in the necessary information.

Be on your way to having some awesome abs, a lean body, and a healthier you. Read the information above and then write down everything that is relevant to you. Modify, adjust, reshape. You can make it happen and be proud of yourself in the end.

Your Belly Fat Goals

Name:

Age:

Height:

Current Weight:

Target Weight:

What Would You Like to Accomplish?

What is your time frame for accomplishing this?

Add your weight amount and the date at the end of each week here:

Date	Weight

My Specific Belly Fat Diet Plan

Just fill in the details of what you'd like to eat during the days indicated. If you want to change it each week, print out a separate copy for different meal plans.

	Breakfast	Lunch	Dinner	Snack #1	Snack #2
Monday					
Tuesday					
Wednesday					
Thursday					
Friday					
Saturday					
Sunday					

Foods I should avoid:

My Specific Belly Fat Exercise Plan

Fill in the specific information for your exercise plan. You can modify the details throughout the weeks if needed. Print out additional exercise plan sheets as you get further on your belly fat loss journey. Make sure to add a day of rest each week. You do not want to overdo it and cause your body to go into distress.

	Cardio	Length/Time	Strength	Length/Time
Monday				
Tuesday				
Wednesday				
Thursday				
Friday				
Saturday				
Sunday				

Feel confident and successful in your journey to lose those extra pounds around your middle. You need to feel good about becoming healthier. Don't get stuck because you do not like your current diet plan, or because the exercise is making you tired. Keep going! You do not want to be one of the thousands who give up. You'll be the one to say that you beat belly fat and feel great!

Use this article as your guide. There are many benefits that come with shedding those pounds, you just have to stay motivated and keep sight of the final goal. Rest, reduce stress, exercise and eat healthy. Watch how quickly you'll decrease the amount of fat in your body and how quickly you'll feel better. .

Good luck on your journey to becoming the best you that you can be!

Chapter 32 - ACCESS TO BONUS VIDEO AND RECIPES

First of all, we'd like to give you a **BIG HEARTY** Thank you for purchasing our book. We strive to offer you the best service possible and certainly hope that we've been able to give you some kind of ***VALUE for your money's worth!***

If you've learned anything or got at least **1 GOOD IDEA** from our book, we kindly ask that you share that with us and leave some feedback.

Your humble feedback will not only help us to push forward with more helpful products to serve you better, but will also help other lovely customers (such as yourself) to make a purchasing decision as each review will be online for **ALL TO SEE!**

Once Again We Thank You for Your Time with Us and We Wish You **GREAT SUCCESS ON YOUR JOURNEY!**

(Just Click on the Link Below or Copy and Enter It in Your URL, then Copy and Paste the Password in the Box)

http://videoreviewteam.com/flat-belly-miracle

Password: flatbelly123

NOTE: Also If you want ***MORE IN DEPTH LESSONS*** on *How You Can Lose Belly Fat* (There is a Link at the Bottom of the Videos Page) ...**Thank You Once Again!**

www.ingramcontent.com/pod-product-compliance
Lightning Source LLC
Chambersburg PA
CBHW070234290526
45789CB00004B/1623